MY LIFE

AS A PANCREAS

Reflections on Raising a Child with Diabetes

A mother chronicles the first few years
of life with her diabetic child.

Illustrations by Gail Machlis

Design by Leticia Castillo

Inquiries should be addressed to:

Priscilla Call Essert
Telephone (510) 459-3935
www.mylifeasapancreas.com

Copies of this book can be purchased through
http://www.lulu.com OR Amazon.com.

First Printing 2006

Printed in USA

ISBN: 978-1-4303-0521-7

Dedicated to Bill, Miles, Byron, and all of the children
and families touched by juvenile diabetes.

THANKS TO

Gail and Leticia for sharing their talents, Jay and Liz for getting me over the hump, Alexis for her editorial help and support, Kim, Julie, and Archana for all of their guidance over the years, and to the Diabetic Youth Foundation and Dr. Mary for helping our family through a tough time. Lastly, to my husband for being a good sport!

CREDITS

Author, Priscilla Call Essert, worked for over twenty years as a classical flutist. In addition to recording and radio work, she held positions in several orchestras such as the Orquesta Filarmónica de la Ciudad de México, the California Symphony, the Marin Symphony, Opera San Jose, and Berkeley Symphony. She was a professor of music at Mills College in Oakland, CA.

Priscilla currently resides in the San Francisco Bay Area with her husband and two children. When not writing, she plays with a Cuban band, performs with classical chamber ensembles, knits rather than meditates, and is always looking for new creative outlets.

Illustrator and cover artist, Gail Machlis, created the daily cartoon panel "Quality Time," which ran for ten years in newspapers across the country. Her work has appeared in numerous publications including *Ms. Magazine, Cosmopolitan, New Woman,* and *The Artists Magazine.* She has one collection of cartoons, *Quality Time and Other Quandaries* published by Chronicle Books. She is currently writing and illustrating children's books and exhibiting her paintings at San Francisco Bay Area galleries.

Designer, **Leticia Castillo**, brings nine years of creative graphic design experience to this project. She has worked on various books for Bay Area writers and organizations. Her work ranges from print to web design. Her work can be viewed at www.leticiacastillo.com.

TABLE OF CONTENTS

PRELUDE TO BECOMING A PANCREAS

February of 2001, Byron started to change so gradually that it wasn't until much later that it was perceptible. First there were the strange moments when he was uncharacteristically lacking in coordination. (Two teeth were knocked out from a really odd fall.) We attributed it to developmental changes. In the Spring, his behavior started to change at school. The teachers reported moments of extreme activity followed by lintense lethargy such that all he could do was lie on the floor and stare into space. This was like nothing we had seen in him before. Coupled with wetting his bed, we began to wonder.

Then there were the moments when he would complain of a stomachache, claim his stomach was upset, and then ask for a candy bar. No candy bars in the house, he opted for devouring six apricots or more in one sitting. After eating the apricots or any other fruit, the stomachache would go away and then he would drink large quantities of water. I began to wonder even more.

June of 2001, I took Byron in for a physical and explained to the doctor all of these things. I asked him if there was something wrong with the amount of fruit Byron was eating, or the volume of water he was drinking. I asked him if the bed wetting might be caused by a bladder infection. The doctor assured me that everything was normal and not to worry. He figured it was probably anxiety over the year ending and that there is no such thing as eating too much fruit. He went so far as to congratulate me on getting him to eat fruit in the first place. I still wondered...

July of 2001, one month later, we headed out on a camping trip. After an evening of barbeque followed by marshmallows and chocolate, the quiet night kept getting interrupted by Byron's frustrated cries for someone to take him to the bathroom. He got up at least 5 times with such an urgent need to urinate that he couldn't even make it to the bathroom. Now we were certain there was a problem. In the morning, we packed up our damp tent and soaked sleeping bags, and headed home.

The drive home took longer than usual as we must have stopped every hour at any location that had a bathroom. After using the restroom, he would complain of being thirsty. We hesitated to give him water, but the need was so intense that we acquiesced. With the feverish dance between thirst and hunting for bathrooms, the drive seemed to take forever. Once we reached home, we phoned the doctor and he asked us to bring him in immediately. My husband, Bill, left with Byron and I stayed back with Miles, our older son.

When Bill called me to tell me that Byron had diabetes and was being admitted to the hospital, I was not that surprised. I was really scared, but not surprised. Somewhere deep inside I knew he had diabaetes but I just couldn't admit it. The signs were the there. The doctor said not to worry. I asked for tests, but the doctor said not to worry. It was staring us in the face, but we hoped it was something else, and chose instead to worry about what that something else might be. It seemed less scary than the alternative. Besides, the doctor told me what I wanted to hear: not to worry.

In retrospect, we were very lucky. There are so many different ways things could have played out. I have heard so many stories of "the diagnosis" and many of them involve comas and much more drama than we experienced.

Even though I had an instinct, the disease seemed to come out of the blue and was followed by a string of questions. Like many others, I wondered if it is was something we did or didn't do, why we didn't catch it earlier...

After a day or so, I let go of the questions. I tended to the soggy camping gear waiting for me on our deck. I applied various ointments to the poison oak I got from frequent night-time walks to the bathroom while on our camping trip, and began transitioning to life as a pancreas.

MOVING ON BUT NOT READY TO TEACH

I hear the diagnosis and I am numb. I don't want to believe it. Will denial reign?

I go through the diabetes training in a fog, I bring my child home from the hospital, and I wonder if I might wake up the next morning and find out it was all a big mistake. I am still numb. Denial seems to reign.

After a couple of days, it becomes quite clear that I am not dreaming and that I am now in charge of life support for my child. In reality, this has always been the case. Being a parent is serious stuff!

At last, I accept the diagnosis. I begin to move forward. I yearn to move forward. But what about those around me? I seem to have sped past them. I feel alone. How do I handle all of the people I meet who know as little about diabetes as I did before Byron was diagnosed? What about all of the people I meet who think they know everything about my child because their aunt or uncle has diabetes—Type II Diabetes—but to them it is all the same. I soon realize that I am adapting, I am moving forward, I am not so numb, but those around me are not traveling through this with me. Strangers and loved ones can't quite catch up. It is lonely.

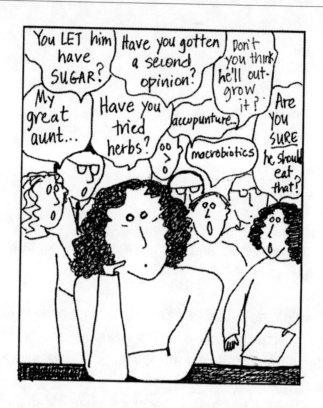

We leave the house—our cocoon where we learned to manage. Managing is a bit harder out in public; people are aghast when I allow him to have sugar. They think sugar is the last thing any diabetic should have. It bothers me, but how can I be angry? I am angry but I don't feel I have the right to be. I mean, I didn't understand the difference before I arrived in this place. I need to be patient. Still, this brings me no comfort. I feel such a gap between where I am and where everyone else is.

Time passes, and the gap doesn't shrink unless I put in a lot of effort. I begin to make peace with this gap as I realize I have some control over it. The gap closes if I educate people. It closes if I explain things quietly and patiently. I begin to see this gap as an opportunity. Still, there are days when I just can't seem to seize the moment to educate and edify the curious ones around me. I know it is my responsibility, and most days I willingly accept that responsibility, but other days I just refuse. I think that's fair. Don't you?

THE DIABETIC IN MY FAMILY

I often hear people describe their children by their main interest or talent. As a child, I was the musician in the family. One of my brothers was the runner, the other brother was the smart one, and my sister was the one who caused trouble. I now have my own children and my son Byron is the diabetic in the family. He is a happy and healthy 10-year-old boy who happens to have diabetes. He was diagnosed with Type I Diabetes just a couple of days after his 6th birthday and his bravery and courage since the diagnosis continue to amaze and inspire me.

Because Byron was diagnosed at such a young age, it is hard to say how much diabetes has changed his life. Are there things he isn't doing that he might have done? Or has the diabetes helped him become who he is? Did diabetes turn him into a voracious reader and a talented writer? Is it because of the diabetes that he is fearless (often to my own chagrin)? I don't know, but I will always wonder.

Byron likes to refer to himself as a boy who happens to have diabetes rather than a diabetic who happens to be a boy. The only thing he hates more than being called a diabetic is when people talk about his disease without including him. He figures it is "his" just like his room is his and his bike is his...His boundaries are clear and he is not afraid to

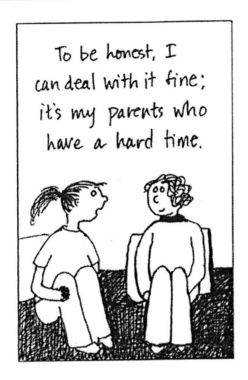

let me know when I have crossed them. I sometimes forget that it is not "my" disease but his: an easy mistake to make when you are acting as someone's pancreas.

Byron likes his privacy, which makes his willingness to let me share my stories with you even more amazing. Even though they are stories from my perspective of life with Byron, they still invade his privacy a bit. Then why would he agree to all of this? He knows better than anyone that grownups are going to have much more trouble coping with their child's diabetes than the kid will, and that they need all the help they can get!

LIFE BEFORE BECOMING A PANCREAS

As private as Byron is, I was raised to be even more private. I grew up in a conservative, suburban New England town in a time when you weren't supposed to admit that you were having troubles or that you needed help, and you certainly never talked about anything going on in the family. You were supposed to suffer in silence, be stoic, smile, and only dwell on the good things in life.

When I was 8 years old, my sister was born with Spina Bifida, and due to several complications she spent a great deal of her childhood in hospitals. My parents struggled to work, raise five kids, and to shuttle the crew between track practice, doctor's offices and hospitals. It took a toll on them and the entire family. Despite all of this, we remained silent and stumbled forward.

When I was in high school, one of my brothers struggled with depression. He left for college and shortly thereafter sank into a deep depression and had to leave school. After several suicide attempts, he succeeded in killing himself in February of 1977. Again, I watched as my parents endured an unfortunate and painful moment in their life. Still, we all remained silent and shared nothing with those around us.

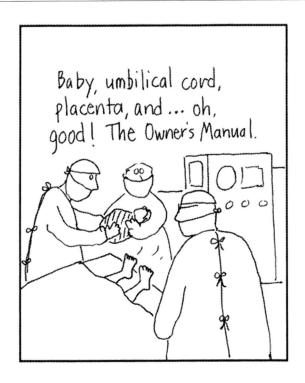

As a young teen, there was little I could do except watch what was going on around me, try to understand it as best I could, continue living my life, and respect my family by remaining silent. I felt rather helpless and I spent a lot of time wishing that someone would come along and help our family pull together, heal, and recover. Help rarely comes if you don't ask for it.

By the time I went to college, I finally got the help I needed. I broke the silence, began sharing my stories with trusted friends, and they in turn shared theirs. I felt years of pain, grief, and sadness slowly dissolve as we opened up and I realized that I wasn't alone: that others have gone through similar things and survived. It turned out to be the most amazing gift I could have given myself as well as others.

The importance of sharing stories became clear to me once again after I had my first child. In my search to find a book that would give me a look into a the journey of motherhood – not just how-to guides – I found a book that not only inspired me, but helped me reconnect with the humor of parenting and taught me to not take myself so seriously. To this day, I know that reading *Operating Instructions* by Anne Lamott, was critical in helping me to make the transition from being childless to being a parent. She gave me the chance to peek into the life of parents, all the mistakes we can and will make, all of the doubts we will have but will move past, and how raising a child will take us places we never imagined we would go.

So what does all of that have to do with writing this book? When Byron was diagnosed with diabetes, I once again felt deep grief and a profound sense of loss, not to mention fear and confusion. I had an intense need to get lost in the tales of others so that I might unearth a nugget that would help me move forward and to make sense of the new place I had arrived. I couldn't find anything at all: no stories to comfort me and little to help me get started on this new journey. I decided that it was time for me to put my own stories down on paper. From that day forward, I jotted down events that I felt were significant points in the adventure of caring for Byron.

Today you have those stones and observations in your hands: a series of significant moments in my life with Byron that I hope will offer you some support, comfort, and maybe a laugh or two.

HOW I BECAME A PANCREAS

My husband and I were at a party that I did not even really want to attend. I was extremely tired after getting up every hour to test Byron's sugar and just wanted to be in bed. We went, I met someone new, and she asked the question that so many of us ask: the and-what-do-you-do -for-a-living-question. I just did not have the energy to be creative or to deliver another mini-lecture that adequately describes all that I juggle. My mind was foggy, I had no idea what to say, yet after a couple of seconds a response just seemed to pop out of me. To this day, I don't know where it came from, but I replied, "I'm a full-time pancreas".

Yes, I really said that to someone. The look on her face was priceless and I would have enjoyed it more had I not shocked myself with my response. It took an altered state of mind brought on by sleep deprivation mixed with a pinch of oh-what-the-hell for me to get to the truth of my life: I am my child's pancreas. That is exactly what you are for a young child with diabetes. You are their pancreas! Another title. I feel so much better.

Before I had children, I worked full time in music. When people asked me what I did for a living I would describe myself as being a professor of music, a concert flutist, a chamber musician, or an

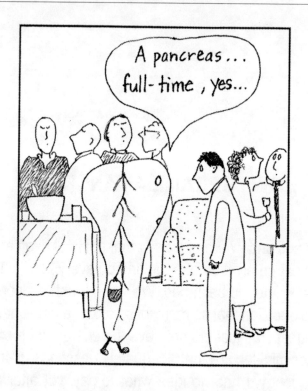

educator. I had titles. Titles are so convenient and simplify answering the dreaded age-old question, "And what's your job?"

After having kids, those titles expanded to "mom" with all prior descriptors still in tact. What did expansion mean? Well, it meant that I had to work faster, sleep a lot less, and that I had to improvise and quickly adjust when my kid's needs would suddenly force me to change plans. Still, I had a title.

Just as I was getting used to being flexible and felt more comfortable with wearing numerous hats, Byron developed Type I Diabetes. Two months later, he was just starting first grade, and there was no such thing as a day with good blood sugar control. We were receiving calls on a daily basis that required one of us to rush to his school to give him an injection or to handle his low blood sugar. Since I was working closer to home and had more flexibility than my husband, it was usually me.

Flexibility aside, the reality was that I had to leave rehearsals, lessons, and concerts...not a good thing in my business. Simply put, my work no longer fit with the rest of my life. Therefore, at the age of 43, I made the decision to stop working for the first time in at least twenty years. This is when I became a pancreas with an identity crisis.

The depth of this identity crisis slowly became apparent to me through the stress I would feel when new acquaintances would ask me what I do for a living. I no longer had a title to throw around that could easily define me in a couple of sentences or less. I could not seem to master the art of answering the question without over-explaining my life, or without sounding or feeling (I am not sure which) a bit defensive. I would deliver an defensive-sounding monologue on how it is much more important to know how someone spends their time than how they earn a living. This was a great way to avoid answering the question, but it was exhausting and I am certain I scared off quite a few people. Shoot, I scared myself. Eventually, sleep deprivation brought the truth out of me. I am now a pancreas.

WHAT DO THE DOCTORS REALLY KNOW?

After Byron was diagnosed, his doctors gave us the most amazing gift. The gift came in the form of advice. Although sleep deprived and nervous about bringing our son home, their advice burnt itself into my memory and I will never forget it because it was so unexpected.

They said that we would end up knowing more about our son's diabetes than all of the experts combined, that we shouldn't be surprised when it happens, that it is perfectly normal, and that it is a healthy side effect of caring for your child.

I thought they were just trying to make us feel better. It occurred to me that it might be the perfect way to get us to leave the hospital and get us out of their hair. I didn't find their advice all that reassuring. I mean, after all, don't we expect doctors to have all the answers? What are they there for if they don't? Although we know it isn't really their job, there is, deep down, an infantile desire for a doctor to know everything and to make things all better.

Almost 3 years later, I can now say they were right. What I know doesn't always make sense, doesn't agree with books or medical wisdom, and doesn't even match up with the experiences of other

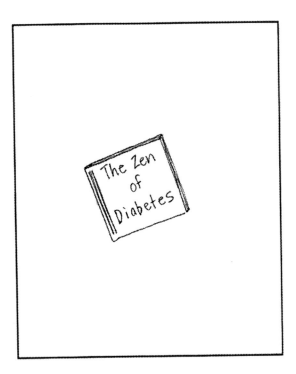

parents of diabetics. What I know is my son's body and his soul.

When he is stressed out, I know what will happen to his blood sugar. I know how quickly a slice of pizza works in his body. I know what happens to his blood sugar if he doesn't sleep enough. I know what happens when we travel and there is a time change. If he is a bit pale, I know whether he is sick or if his sugar is low even before I test.

You can't find this stuff in a book and you can't get it from a doctor. This is what I like to call the art of diabetes. I guess you could get a bit cheeky and call it the Zen of Diabetes Management...all those variables in your child's life that you can't control and that don't fit on the charts, but you know they happen and you know they are real. You can calculate your child's carbohydrate ratio, his insulin sensitivity, and then try to plug that into every situation. That is the science. Then, there is the art: all the variables for which there are no formulas or hard science. Doctor's, unless they are themselves diabetics, don't know a lot about the art. Diabetic doctor or not, you are now the translator for your child's body.

I like to think of the art of diabetes management as everything that goes into the memo or comment section of the diabetes logbook. A lot of doctors don't pay much attention to the memo section – they are not necessarily equipped to handle this part of your child's care. They aren't there to discuss the subtleties of your child's illness. It is much easier to talk about the science – concrete issues – rather than intangibles: carbohydrate ratios, A1C readings, kidney function, insulin pumps, the latest insulin etc.

I know my child's body inside out and I have answers that no doctor will ever have. Doctors cheer us on, are a great support team, are a great resource, and I can't imagine caring for Byron without them, but the bottom line is that I am now an interpreter of my son's body. I translate his body into terms understood by those in science, and without this sort of input, Byron's health would be compromised. I am thankful that his doctors have healthy egos that make room for this sort of partnership.

HOW MUCH CAN GO WRONG?

If I indulge myself, I can worry about so many things. I am really good at it! Want me to prove it? Let's see, I can worry about the things that the specialists say will probably happen as my son ages. I can worry about the things they say might happen but they aren't sure yet because there hasn't been enough testing done to prove it. Worse yet, I can worry that there is something that will go wrong that nobody knows about because it simply hasn't happened to anyone as of yet. For instance, if my child gets a bloody nose, will he bleed longer than a child without diabetes? I know, it sounds ridiculous, but I wonder about these things. How much can go wrong?

My son sometimes plays goalie for his team, the Weasels. (Contrary to their name they are a kick-butt soccer team.) Byron is an aggressive and fearless player and when a ball comes his way, he will do what it takes to block it. In one game, a ball comes his way, he makes an amazing stop, but unfortunately, his nose does most of the work. His first reaction is joy and ecstasy. This reaction is quickly replaced by panic as he wipes his nose, sees blood all over his glove, and plentiful streaks of blood on his jersey. He drops the ball, runs towards me with arms outstretched, tears now mixing with a torrent of blood, and his white sport shirt turning deep red before my eyes. The coach rips off his

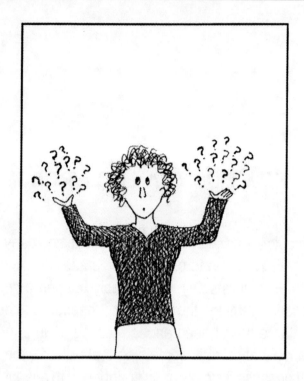

shirt to give it to my son as no tissue in the world is going to handle this bloody flood. My heart races and my focus is totally on him as I catch his blood and try to speak in a calm and reassuring manner while other parents freak out. What is my first thought?

As I stare at the blood soaked items around me, I wonder if a diabetic bleeds more than other kids. I mean, will it stop? Could he hemorrhage? Is there something in the training manual that I missed? Will his blood sugar plummet as a result of the trauma or will it soar? Will he ever stop bleeding? How do I check his sugar while I am holding a mountain of Kleenex over his face. Ah, I have it, I can test the sugar from his bleeding nose...that would be efficient!

Finally, I let go of all of that craziness and just hold my son. Did

I worry about a broken nose or his ego? No, I wondered if a diabetic bleeds more than other kids. Stranger things have happened. There is so much to know and so much that no one tells you. There is also so much I know that they don't know.

They don't know how much his toes ache when they get cold and that his toes get cold so much faster than my other son, Miles, who does not have diabetes. Is it possible that he had chicken pox three times and still had no immunity because he was about to become a diabetic? When he gets a cough, it sounds much worse than anyone I know. Is this the diabetes?

To prevent myself from going crazy, I try to strike a balance between what I know to be true about the workings of my son's body, trust my instincts, look at the medical facts, and then go from there.

WHO IS THE EXPERT IN YOUR FAMILY?

Every couple I know has someone who is great at cooking and someone who isn't, someone who can handle the finances and someone who can barely add. Most couples balance each other out in one way or another. In our family, I am the one who usually deals with the kids when they are sick. My husband, Bill, has a difficult time accepting illness in himself as well as others. I am accustomed to illness and find it rather gratifying to take care of my family members when they are under the weather. So, when the boys get the flu or a cold, I take care of them. If they wake up in the middle of the night with a fever or a stomach bug, I sit with them for as long as it takes to get them to sleep. I sometimes complain, but the truth is that it works for me—works for us—as long as I can occasionally complain and Bill listens.

When Byron was first diagnosed, Bill surprised me by insisting that he be the one to stay at the hospital. He went to the hospital with Byron and stayed the first night while I spent time with Miles and tried to find someone to care for him so that I could get to the hospital the next day. (Without any family living nearby this was no easy task.) When I finally arrived at the hospital, Bill was ready to jump out of his skin. Twenty-four hours of watching Byron get poked and prodded, dealing with doctors and nurses, and trying to master the basics of diabetes care left him a wreck. As soon as I arrived, I could tell that he desperately needed a break. We stayed together a while, and then he returned home while I had my training and passed the time watching numerous episodes of Sponge Bob with Byron.

Another day passed, and Byron and I returned home from the hospital. Over the next few days, Bill and I both struggled to remember proper techniques for mixing insulin, giving an injection, and timing Byron's food intake with his insulin. It was extremely overwhelming for both of us. We were painfully aware that our child's life was in our hands in a way we hadn't quite thought about prior to the diagnosis. I noticed Bill was having much more trouble remembering things than I was. Afraid of making mistakes or of hurting Byron, he quickly passed certain duties my way.

Bill returned to work the day after Byron returned home. Alone and without anyone to check in with other than doctors, I had to learn to trust myself, and I had to quickly learn to care for Byron and to develop competency. There wasn't anyone around to consult with. I got up frequently to check Byron's sugar, I lived and breathed insulin/carb ratios and I had charts for everything. I attended the clinic appointments, started developing a relationship with the diabetes team, and through that team found a lot of support.

Little by little, Bill's involvement changed. My sense of competency grew at about the same rate as his declined. He felt less and less confident in mixing insulin and determining insulin doses. He couldn't seem to grasp the ratios, was always checking in with me before he made any determination, and then it hit me: I had become "the expert"—something I hadn't intended to be. I had a feeling we were in trouble. I didn't think it was wise to have one expert. I thought there should be two.

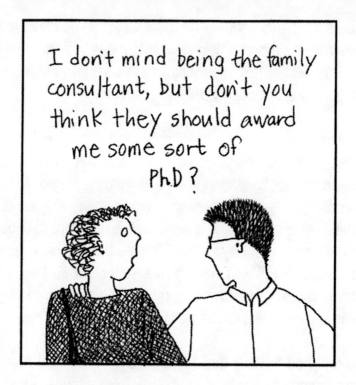

One year after Byron was diagnosed, it was still clear that I was the consultant for Byron's health. Bill was a fabulous helper, but I was tired of having only a helper rather than a full partner. It didn't seem like a good thing for me, for Byron, or for our relationship. Looking for answers and support, I brought my two children to Bearskin Meadow Camp (sponsored by the Diabetic Youth Foundation of Concord, CA), a camp for children with diabetes and their families. I went hoping to meet other families, children with diabetes, and to refresh my skills and add new ones. I wanted to see if my husband and I could change the direction in which we were heading.

After talking with many families and children at the camp, I realized that most families have an expert. It seems to be the nature of it all. It isn't such a "bad" thing. Actually, it is rather efficient. In fact, it seems that when both parents try to be the expert, the care isn't necessarily any better and you end up with two tired and stressed out parents rather than one.

My husband helps out quite a bit, but many of the details are hard for him. The management of this disease isn't one my husband's strengths. He has a difficult time with the ratios; I thrive on them. He can't handle the intangibles such as the normal curve of insulin which isn't really all that normal. I live for intangibles. He can't handle the number of variables (most of which are uncontrollable) that affect diabetes control such as growth spurts, stress, exercise, fat content of a food, illness. If I don't have enough variables, I am miserable. This diabetes thing isn't concrete enough for him. He knows when he is in over his head and knows when to ask for help and how to accept it. It's o.k.

Bearskin Meadow gave me four peaceful days in the woods, new friends, new perspectives, peace of mind, a new look at how my marriage functions, and the knowledge that Byron will be just fine if his mom continues to be the diabetes consultant for his dad. His dad will be really happy knowing that his wife will no longer try to make him an expert. His mom will be a lot easier to live with now that she accepts where she is. Thank you Bearskin Meadow!

FROM SUGAR NAZI TO SUGAR-PUSHING MOMMA

When my oldest son, Miles, was born in 1994, I was determined to keep his diet as pure as possible. I made baby food, I made bread, I bought organic produce, avoided refined foods and so many more things that in retrospect were a bit over the top. I was NEVER going to let refined sugar touch his lips. Was it living in Berkeley or was it a reaction to having had too much of that amazing white bread that you could roll up into a ball and spit through a straw? Who knows? Whatever the reason, I maintained this degree of diligence until preschool started and then the real world came crashing in. Enter Ding Dongs, Ho Ho's, Oreos, Twinkies and more.

Now let us fast forward a few years to 2001, the year that Byron was diagnosed with Type I Diabetes. This was a huge turning point in our lives—the time that our cupboards began to house life savers, sugar cubes, hard candies, juice with no pulp (a much better sugar high than with pulp) and many other sources of "fast" sugar.

It happened slowly, but before long I found myself in the aisle of Pack & Save with a cart overflowing with every type of fast sugar I could get my hands on. I needed to be prepared for unexpected visits from hypoglycemia. As I would stash sugar in every place I might find my son having a low, I wondered if this is how a squirrel feels as it prepares for winter.

By now, diabetes is pretty integrated into our lives. Sometimes things can get so integrated into your life that you begin to think of it as normal. Every once in a while, I have an incident that reminds me that relative to the lives of others, our lives are not "normal".

Parties (with kids) are always stressful for us. It is difficult to keep track of everything that Byron eats. Kids don't stand in one place long enough to really get an idea of what is going into their bodies. They don't remember what they ate or how much (so much for carbohydrate counting), they forget if they corrected for their food, you forget if your spouse corrected for their food, and on and on. Blood glucose goes really high and then really low. You know, the ping-pong dilemma. It's crazy!

At one parent/child gathering, my son is running around all over the yard, he begins to feel very low, and comes to me for help. I excuse myself from a conversation, test his sugar, get him a bit of juice, and decide that he should have a cookie to give him a bit of extra fuel to safely run on. It feels like a pit stop where you have to guesstimate input, output, and the energy required to make it to the end of the race. You don't want to run out of fuel in the middle of Nebraska do you?

I return to the group of people I had been talking with, I resume the conversation as if nothing has happened. (I have become quite adept at this.) At this point, my son runs up to me, thrusts half of his cookie and his test kit into my hands while I am talking, and happily runs off. It takes me a moment to realize that once again I have become his pack mule. Another few seconds pass and I realize that I am holding his half-eaten cookie – his fuel!

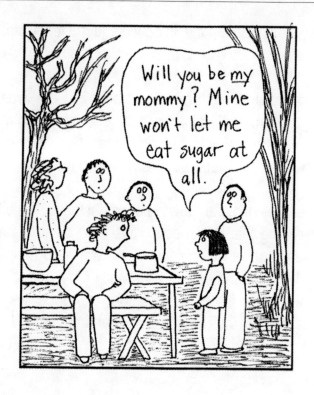

Do I run after him? No time for that. Do I calmly call for him? No, too frightened. What do I do? With no regard for the ears of those near me, I yell across the yard with the most amazing projection. The words that come out of my mouth make me wonder how the sugar Nazi in me has been taken over by the sugar dealer. Here is the treachery that I speak: "Byron, get back here now and finish this cookie. You can't play unless you finish this cookie. You MUST have sugar. If you don't get back here now you will be in time-out!" Then it happens – a silence more deafening than my screams.

I look around and my friends have stopped talking and are staring at me, their jaws hanging open. Here it is again, the moment when you realize that your life is so amazingly different from those around you. Some of these folks didn't know about Byron's diabetes and thought I was just out of my mind. Others knew about it, but forgot, and don't really understand it enough to make sense of this sugar dealer yelling in their ears. Others think they know about it and believe that the sugar is his problem and that if we get rid of it he would be fine and perhaps cured. What do I do? Do I remain silent? Do I become a walking public service announcement and seize an opportunity to educate?

I didn't have to make a choice. Something quite serendipitous occurred that brought humor and levity to the situation. A little girl came up to me, pulled on my slacks, and said, "Would you be my mommy? My mommy won't let me have sugar." Saved by the girl! Who would have guessed that my role as the mother of a child with diabetes would make me sought after as a mommy!

As for my friends, they recovered. They were actually amused and oddly grateful. They were grateful to have a peek into my life with Byron. The disease he has is so invisible to them. He looks fine. He acts fine (most of the time). He never complains. I rarely complain. They don't understand the work that goes into keeping him stable. How could they? (I wish they could know, but if they knew, they would be in my shoes, and that wouldn't be great.) A normal event in our life, shared in public for all to witness, gave our friends a chance to understand us a little better.

FROM SUICIDE TO ICE CREAM

I lost a brother to suicide when I was 18. So, when Byron, at the ripe age of seven, declared that he wanted to kill himself, you can imagine that it might have pushed a few buttons.

It's moments like these that I am grateful for having read – or even inhaled – several books on child rearing and child psychology. It is moments like these that I am grateful for having been in therapy for a few years. It is times like these that I am grateful for having taken yoga! Here is the story...

I picked my son up from school and we had a rare moment alone without his big brother. He seemed a little down and I asked him how he was. He was silent for a few seconds and then said, "I want to kill myself". My mind started spinning as I tried to figure out all the reasons why he would want to do this to himself. My mind still racing, I took a few yoga breaths and calmly said, "O.k. It is your body and you can do what you want with it, but we would really miss you and would feel really sad for a really long time". Silence....

Then he said that he hates his name and he wants to change it. I told him that would be fine and asked what his new name would be. He said that he wanted to be Zorro Call Essert. I assured him that he could

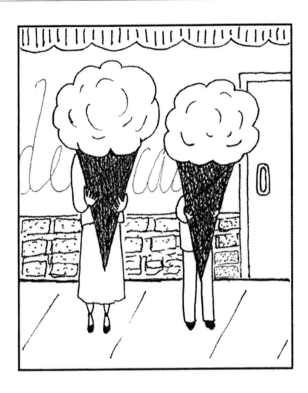

change his name to Zorro if he would like and that I would be happy to bring him to City Hall to fill out the necessary papers.

When I said his new name out loud, he went on another path and said, "I actually like my name, but I hate having diabetes." I told him that I could understand this and he should tell me everything he hates about it and get it all out right now. At this, he moaned, whined, cried a bit, and then he said, "Actually, all I really want is to get some ice cream."

Now, hold your judgment! After that type of conversation and all the tricks my mind played on me, I was exhausted. My will power had been worn down. We went and had ice cream; He laughed, smiled, and thanked me profusely and said he had just had a rotten day. You could say it was manipulation, but I don't think so. I think it was a kid who had just had enough, and somewhere on that path from suicide

31

to ice cream I finally got to hear some of his real feelings and internal struggles about having diabetes. It was the first time – in one whole year – that he had complained about having diabetes. In that moment, I trusted my instincts, and decided that it was more important to park the car, shut off the phone, hang out, let him vent, give him the ice cream, and to help him get back to feeling better about his life.

We entered Baskin Robbins, he selected his ice cream, and he willingly took an injection. His sugar was a bit out of whack for a while, but it was all worth it to hear—for the first time ever—his deepest feelings about having diabetes, to see a smile return to his face, and to see a look of relief gradually replace a tortured, terrified look as he slowly unburdened himself.

He didn't even finish the ice cream. It wasn't about the ice cream...

DARE TO TRAVEL

Before having kids, I used to be able to travel with one carry on bag. Packing list? Never! When our kids were born I began to understand the evolution of the packing list. I also began to understand those weary parents I used to snicker at as they lugged the diaper bag, the stroller, the car seats and the screaming kids onto the plane. I never imagined it would be me—that I would one day be staring enviously at carefree young adults breezing through the airport as I attempt to juggle baby cargo, temper tantrums, and snack boxes.

In due time our kids reached a point where they could carry their own bags. Their plane toys were replaced by a good book or a few word puzzles. The security blanket or favorite bear was replaced by a pack of gum and a favorite pen and pad for doodling. Ahh, what a life...

Our newly acquired ease of traveling quickly changed when Byron was diagnosed. Shortly after the diagnosis, we traveled from San Francisco to London. This was in December, 2001. With all of the heightened security measures that were put into place after September 11, we couldn't help wondering how we were going to get syringes and vials of insulin on the plane when you couldn't even carry nail clippers. What could we take on the plane and what would we need? Did we need a note from a doctor? The questions kept coming and I didn't seem to find the answers in the books I was reading.

I set about scouring government travel advisories, diabetes websites, airline resources and more looking for advice on how to travel with a diabetic. Although I found some helpful tips, most of the information was far too general and/or ambiguous. As with many things, what I really needed to know I learned by getting out there and just doing it.

Since the trip to England in 2001, we have traveled extensively in the United States, Europe, and Mexico. What follows are eight things to consider:

1. Don't ever voluntarily disclose your child's diabetes. Some airlines suggest that you call ahead to let them know you have a diabetic child with you. Others ask you to disclose this information upon check-in. Don't do it! We did it and it really wasn't a good idea. It leads to long delays and more questions than anyone should have to answer. If they notice the syringes and insulin or are stumped by the insulin pump, then whip out a note from your doctor. More often than not they notice the fingernail clipper that I forgot to remove from my purse or they want to pull apart every part of my flute case. (This never ceases to amaze me.) Occasionally, you get surprised. On a recent trip to Italy, the inspectors in Pisa were quite suspicious about the things we were carrying and did ask us for a doctor's note.

I had almost left it home as it had been ages since anyone asked for it. I was glad I had packed it.

2. Travel with insulin vials inside the original package whether or not the package has been opened. It might get you through any inspection faster than a copy of the prescription. Still, you might want to allow an extra half hour to check-in. On a trip to Oaxaca, Mexico, a wickedly curious security person in San Francisco spent 30 minutes checking every box of insulin, every bottle of test strips, and every infusion set. The same was true for a return trip from London. They seemed to have so much fun with the task. Who would have guessed?

3. Never pack your supplies in a bag that will be checked. Place all of your diabetes supplies in a bag that can fit in the overhead compartment. Don't place them under the seat. We once placed everything under the seat, it was stepped on, and all of the infusion sets and syringes were damaged.

4. Find out how you can order supplies if for some reason you lose your supplies or they are stolen. This is critical for pumpers as pumping supplies are not readily available. This step is crucial when traveling out of the country. We had a very accomplished doctor in Spain who had never, ever seen an insulin pump. Not a good omen!

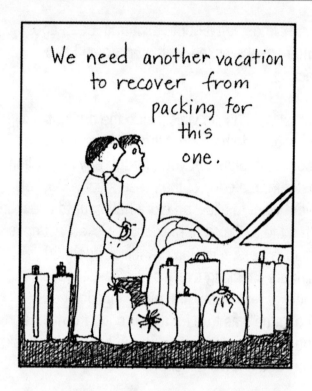

5. Familiarize yourself with medical facilities in the area you will be visiting. You don't want to try to find a place at 2:00 a.m. when nobody is around to help you. Of course, we have never had a diabetic emergency while traveling. Rather, we have had sliced hands, almost severed limbs... The bloody stuff!

6. Not every place you travel to will have a store open when you need it. We spent a month in Oaxaca, Mexico and learned this the hard way. If your child gets sick in the middle of the night, can't chew any food, and you need a ginger ale or Popsicle to help with lows, you can't just

run out to the local market. You do have to think
ahead. A bit of disaster planning goes a long way.

7. If you are a pumper, don't pre-fill reservoirs.
   The reservoirs end up being useless as they just
   develop bubbles over the course of the trip. The
   bubbles are fun to look at, but aren't so good for
   your kid!

8. We used to worry about Byron going low on a plane
   flight. We rarely worried that he would go high.
   However, high blood sugar is more likely. Lack of
   activity alone will cause higher blood sugar readings. Then there is the food issue. Airline fare
   such as pretzels, chips, crackers, and more can
   really wreak havoc on blood sugar. Byron rarely
   eats the meals and lives on the snacks which are
   loaded with fat. It is a good idea to have some
   low-carb or carb-free food with you. Have plenty
   of options for highs, not just lows. You don't want
   to have an inactive, hungry kid with high sugar
   on your hands. Trust me when I say this is not a
   great combination!

Although traveling with a diabetic child might seem daunting, it
gets easier with time. It requires a bit more planning, an extra bag or
two, a little extra patience, and a sense of humor. The adventures you
will have far outweigh the rest of it.

A NEW SCHOOL YEAR:
MORE THAN A NEW LUNCH BOX AND
BIGGER BACKPACK

While other parents cannot wait for each new school year to begin, I have to say that I dread it. The beginning of school means it is time to start putting together the year's 504 Plan. What is a 504 Plan? A 504 plan is a legal document designed to outline a program of instructional services to help students with special needs are in a regular education setting. The 504 Plan falls under the provisions of the Rehabilitation Act of 1973.

About mid-August, the school sends me a blank 504 Plan in the mail. I am supposed to know exactly what to put down on this form, but my mind feels as blank as the page. How do I explain my child's needs to the school? Diabetes care is an art—not just a science—and it creates all sorts of situations that require instinct and a deep knowledge of your child's body. Like most forms, the 504 Plan does not acknowledge gray areas and leaves no room for "if-this-then-that" scenarios. It demands concrete answers to things that are far from concrete. Still, I have to get it together, so how do I do it?

By the end of August, I start to notate every morsel of food that enters my child's body and its impact on his blood sugar so that I am sure that his carbohydrate/insulin ratios have not changed (how much insulin it takes to bring his sugar down 100 points and how many carbohydrates it takes to bring his sugar up 100 points). Although I watch his food intake, I begin to back off from other aspects of his diabetes care to see how much he can do for himself. I say back off, but I am still watching everything while trying to make it seem like I'm not. (You would have to ask him how well I pull this off.) Can he really do his own site change? Can he still give himself a shot? Can he still draw a syringe? Checklist in hand, I feel like a hovering, neurotic, anxiety-ridden mom, and I barely recognize myself. I don't like having to monitor him like this. It begins to feel like he is a lab experiment, and I resent this. But how else do you establish a plan that works?

During the summer, I am able to see most of what Byron eats, have more control over snacks and meals, and can more easily plan for exercise. As a result, his blood sugars are more stable. Even if they are not stable, at least I have a better idea as to why. When school starts, no matter how I draft the 504 Plan, I lose control and Byron's blood sugars are much more volatile. I can try to create some control through the 504 plan, but the reality is that it never feels like you have enough control. It is tough to let go!

Each new school year is a new lesson in letting go of my child. If I give him complete responsibility for his homework and he fails, we can fix it pretty easily. If I give him complete responsibility for his diabetes care and he fails, that could be a really big problem. When he started 3rd grade I decided it was time to include him in the process. It takes a few days of negotiating with him to figure out what he is comfortable doing and then to compare that to what I think he can do or

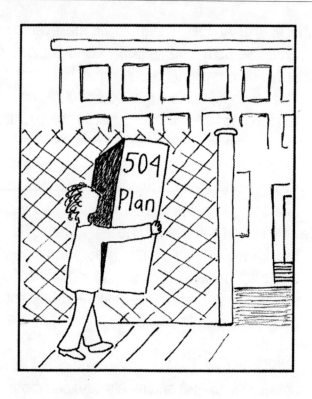

should do. What sort of safety net does he need? How much watching over does he need? What accountability should he have? We hash it out and the plan starts to take shape. Now we wait for the staff training day.

Staff training day arrives and I march into the meeting with a box of spare supplies for the office, a low box for the classroom, an instruction packet for substitutes, and the 504 plan in hand. The principle, the district nurse, an aid, and a few other interested folks gather around the table. We look at the plan and notice a few gaps. When is physical education? Can he handle having a late lunch? Will he have a test kit in his desk or in the hallway? Then there is talk of the disaster plan. What do we do in the event of earthquake or some other disaster? If an earthquake demolishes the office, how can we get to his insulin supply...how...what if...how...what if...

As the discussion continues, I take a brief moment to look up and around the room, and what I see are some faces starting to cloud over. I see my own fear mirrored in those faces. I see doubt and I hear the silent question burning in all of us: how do you really prepare for everything and anything? How do you plan for every possible scenario? You can't. You can try, but you really can't plan for everything. Anything can happen and there is never a guarantee that you will be ready or prepared. You train staff, you train your friends, you stash sugar and insulin wherever you can, and then you cross your fingers and hope that all works out. You plan, let go, and hope that some very brave and courageous person is around your child if things go wrong.

FROM THE MOUTHS OF BABES:
HOW DO YOU KNOW YOU HAVE
TRAINED EVERYONE WELL?

The 504 Plan is now in place and school starts. Each year, Byron likes me to visit his class to do a brief presentation on diabetes. Sometimes he feels like helping and other times he wants to be more in the background, but either way a presentation is made. He figures the presentation gets all of the information out and all of the questions answered at one time.

Byron insists that I let the kids know that he is just like them except that his pancreas has gone on early retirement. Really, if you think about it, that's all that has happened. The rest of the body is still working just fine except for that lazy old pancreas. Kids enjoy thinking of it this way. It's less scary.

Afraid of having a low and not recognizing it, Byron really wants his buddies to know what to look for. He wants them to understand that when he is low, he might get a little confused, cry more easily, get frustrated more quickly, and that he might say some really mean things and get a bit out of control. He is a fast runner, and he wants them to understand that if he can't run, that is another sign that he is not doing well.

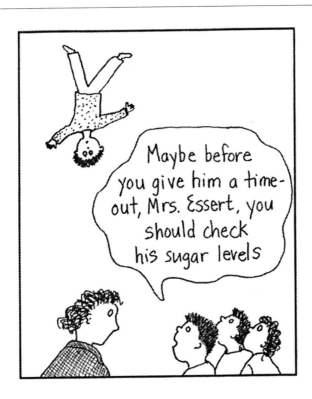

The overall message is this: If Byron is acting like a jerk—something he doesn't usually do unless is sugar is off—before you take it personally, yell at him, tattle on him, or tell him off, point out his behavior to him and suggest he test. If he is high or low, help him take care of it. If he is in target, then you can let him have it! It's a lot to ask of kids, but this is the message he likes to convey. Does it work? Does the message get through?

One day, I am running a meeting for Byron's Cub Scout den and he starts to get really out of control. He is jumping off of tables, yelling, speaking complete nonsense, and being really disruptive while all of his den buddies sit quietly and watch his craziness. I tell him he has to get it together or he will be in a time out. Rather than calming down, he gets progressively worse, so I give him the time out. (Isolation usually works with him.) This doesn't improve things at all. Then I tell him that the meeting will end and I will have to take him home if he can't control himself.

At this point, one of his friends says, "Mrs., Essert, didn't you say that when Byron gets crazy like this that you should test first and then correct his sugar if it is off before you put him in time out?". He was right. I did teach that. I couldn't believe he remembered it. I couldn't believe that I didn't. I felt simultaneously triumphant and stupid.

Clearly, I was successful in getting his friends to understand what he needs and yet I myself did not take my own advice. I was so busy being a den leader that I failed to think like his mom. I was so afraid of the meeting getting out of control that I lost touch with everything I know about Byron.

This experience gave me a bit of insight into how things might play out in the classroom when a teacher is trying to control a class and one kid is going berserk – even if that kid can't help himself.

So how did it turn out? I admitted that I was so wrong, took him out of time out, tested, and guess what? His blood sugar was 55. Boy was that den proud of themselves. We snacked, laughed about it a bit, and then moved on. It was a great meeting and I felt certain that his buddies would be able to spot anything during school. Very reassuring!

LIFE AS A WALKING PUBLIC SERVICE ANNOUNCEMENT

Since the diagnosis, our family has made an effort to participate in the Walk for the Cure sponsored annually by the Juvenile Diabetes Research Foundation. It usually occurs in October, so we begin thinking about fundraising in the spring. We knit things and sell them, bake things and sell them, make lemonade and sell that, and then there is the usual begging for money with nothing at all to sell. Asking for money has always been tough for me, so we usually try to offer a product to sell.

One spring, I was selling baked goods at Byron's school. The lemon bars, cakes, and brownies had sold, and just a few gently picked over treats remained along with lots of crumbs. As I began to pack up our things, a woman approached our homespun operation and bought up our remaining items. As she handed over her spare change, she launched a surprise attack; she began to chastise me for selling sweets for a cause that indicates sweets are forbidden. How did I respond? I didn't know what to say. Clearly she was confused by what type of diabetes my son has. If we had been talking about the same type of diabetes, she would have known that sugar is—at times—life support for my child. Although she was confused and I felt under siege, I

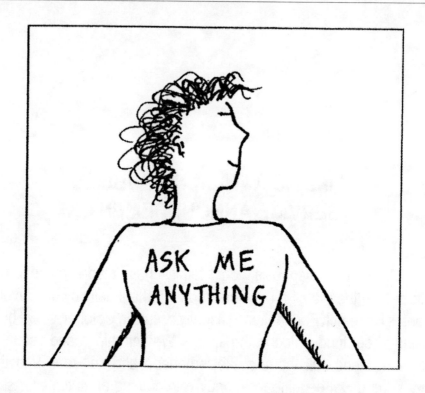

appreciated that she spoke her mind and that she tried to reach out to me.

I now appreciate every person that reaches out to me whether it is out of curiosity, to criticize, to share their stories of relatives who have cured themselves by taking an herb or changing their diet, or to find out when my son will grow out of his illness. I appreciate the store owner who will run for a Coke as my child lies on a store floor with a blood sugar of 26. I appreciate the flight attendants who will hand me sugar even though they question his need for it. I thank all of the people who insist I seek a second opinion to make sure he really has diabetes. Usually, I am annoyed by having to constantly explain myself, but I feel grateful.

When people reach out in this way, they are handing me a golden opportunity to educate, to raise awareness, to connect, and to give a face to this incurable disease. I suppose to some I sound like a walking public service announcement and perhaps a bit preachy at times, and maybe even a tad boring. Too bad! I willingly accept the job.

It isn't such a bad job if it makes my child and every other diabetic safer when they are at school, playing with a friend, on the soccer field, or on a field trip. It isn't such a bad job to have if makes people think about putting the JDRF, DYF, or other organizations that serve diabetics in their will or in their budget. I get to be a change agent. How cool is that?

And what about the woman at the bake sale? Eventually, I came up with a response to her comments. Choosing to keep it simple, I told her that her that sweets are not at all forbidden but that timing is everything. I think that was all she could handle at the moment and she seemed satisfied. I felt like I scored one point on behalf of all of the type one diabetics out there who like to have a cookie now and then and to enjoy it in peace.

PONDERINGS

PONDERING #1
PUMPING: EASIER OR JUST DIFFERENT?

I am always quite amused when I hear parents who want to get a child onto a pump because it will be easier for everyone. It is most certainly easier for the child—especially at school—but it is a lot of work for a parent when their child is not yet in complete control of his or her diabetes care. Even if he is in control during the day, nothing replaces the parents job at night, and that is when things can go really wrong very quickly.

When your child is on the pump you have to monitor blood sugar levels even more than before. You need to program the pump...you need to program and program some more...you have to determine basal rates...you have to think for the pancreas...still more programming...the cord is pinched...no insulin going in to his body... sugar rises faster...is it the pump or is it the site? He rolls over a lot when he sleeps and the site pulls out. Higher blood sugars...More questions and more actions to be taken.

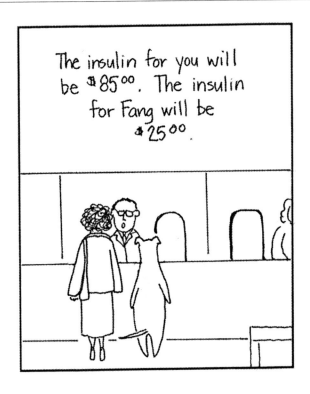

Still, it is all worth it. For once, your child can eat what he wants when he wants. The natural call of hunger rules rather than the normal curve of insulin. Is it less work? No. Is it better? Absolutely!

PONDERING #2
WHAT IS THE REAL COST OF INSULIN?:
THE DARK SIDE OF MEDICINE

I had the most amazing conversation with someone the other day. Her mother has suffered from diabetes for years. She lives alone, is on a fixed income, and struggles to pay the standard $85.00 (more or less) per vial of insulin. So far, not such an exceptional story. We all know someone struggling to pay for their syringes, insulin, and strips.

This same woman happens to own a cat. Her cat gets sick, she brings the cat into the vet, and the cat is diagnosed with diabetes. The vet prescribes insulin; the same exact insulin that this woman is taking. Cost? $25.00 per vial. The volume is the same, the mix is the same, but the cost is staggeringly different.

"How is this possible?, the woman asks of the vet. The vet chalks it up to the greed of pharmaceutical companies.

How is this possible? We all know the medical system isn't working, but I don't think you really knows how bad it is until you develop a desperate need for medicine, and then see the reality of how our medical care gets determined by the insurance we have or by not having it at all. How will all of this influence my son's future? What happens if he can't find a job that provides medical coverage? Will he be able to be self-employed or will that door be closed to him because he will be uninsurable? If he has to pay for everything out of pocket, will he too have to ration his insulin at the expense of his health? I suppose if he really gets desperate, he can buy a cat or dog, hope they are diabetic, and resume a proper insulin regimen at the expense of his pets.

JUST A REGULAR KID

Like many parents, after the birth of my children I was determined to record every milestone of their lives in a special book. I wrote with no purpose in mind except to record my observations and to put together something fun for them to look at when they are older—something tangible from their childhood. As life got busier, I wrote less and less until I wrote no longer.

Recently, I had to spend about a week at home recovering from an illness. I stumbled upon the memory books and decided to read them looking forward to a brief walk down memory lane. In particular, I spent a lot of time looking at Byron's book.

What follows is an abbreviated version of the various milestones in the life of my son Byron. What do you see?

- Finally eating solid food

- Finally crawling

- Now walking and really mobile.

- Starting to potty train and is really competing with big brother.

- Potty training complete (more or less).

- Lost his first tooth (actually, he knocked it out).

- Rode a bike without training wheels.
  Needs to learn to stop!

- Lost another tooth – knocked it out again!

- Off to Kindergarten and couldn't wait to go.

- Starting to read and learning not to hit other kids.

- Teachers reporting behavior changes, weepy, tired, then hyper. Wondering if he has ADHD.

- Fourth of July, 6th birthday, parade in town, big party at our house, huge cake, candy, oh my...

- 6th of July, in the hospital. Diagnosed with diabetes.

- First solo finger poke.

- Another tooth gone. This one fell out on its own.

- Finally allows us to give him an injection in the stomach.

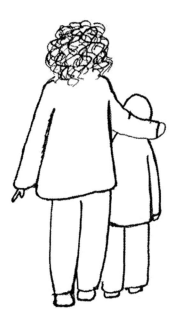

• Thought he was Superman and tried leaping off a wall and cut open his chin. No stitches needed, just glue.

• First blood draw where he didn't nearly bite my finger off.

• First grade starts, and leaving him in the hands of others nearly defeats me.

• First scary low (26) and I grabbed any food in the store I could find, sat on the floor of the store and fed this child! Kids thought this was hilarious (after the fact). Store owners received a bit of education from mom about Type I diabetes. Lot's of

free Coke and yucky carbohydrate things
went down Byron's throat. I sweat a lot.
So, wear deodorant and carry sugar at all times.

• First pump and Byron struggles with where to put
it when sleeping. Will it strangle him? Will it pull
out if he rolls around too much? Does it REALLY work
or is it pure voodoo?

• Stung by several bees today. Freaks out whenever he
sees one! Life outside is far too stressful.

• Byron changed a pump site all by himself, scores his
first goal at soccer game and is quite excited by both,
but mostly by the goal.

Did you catch it? Do you see what I see? One moment I was
charting loss of teeth and the special yet typical milestones of growing
older, and then quite naturally, without even trying, a whole new set
of milestones started creeping in—Byron's unique, one-of-a-kind, huge
steps toward becoming an independent, healthy child who happens to
have diabetes. Life didn't stop after the diagnosis. The teeth kept falling
out, school continued, and his diabetes is part of our life,
but it has not become our life—it is integrated into our life.

Byron certainly has a few more things to manage and organize
than other children, and he definitely has a few extra concerns relating
to diabetes, but all in all, he is just a regular kid. Now that calls for a
celebration! Who would have guessed that regular could have such a
wonderful ring to it?

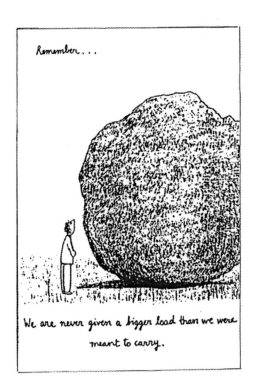

Remember...

We are never given a bigger load than we were meant to carry.

ADDICTED TO CARE GIVING, PART ONE

As I toss and turn the night before my flight to Connecticut I keep trying to figure out the source of my deep anxiety. I am both filled with giddy excitement over the prospect of a night's sleep with my internal worry system turned off, and the lightness that comes from not having to diagnose, calculate, wonder, worry. Then why is it that such a welcome break brings with it so much anxiety? Why is it that the night before I leave I begin to understand that what I am doing is a big job? As exhausting and stressful as it can be to care for Byron, and as many times as I yearn for a break, I am addicted to this role. So many questions and I don't believe that I have a lot of answers.

At 5:00 am I creep into Byron's room. I rub my nose in his soft hair, inhale his scent and hope to memorize it. I feel so sad and scared for him. What if something happens to me on this trip? Have I taught him well? Will he live a long, healthy life?

I leave for a restful vacation with Miles, my oldest son, hoping to have some quality time with this budding teenager. I take deep, long breaths hoping for all of the anxiety to gradually disappear, or to at least become more bearable. Perhaps so called restful vacations are more about having a chance to fall apart and rebuild rather than about feeling "great". If I have a chance to fall apart and regroup, maybe then I can return home to resume a life filled with all sorts of anxieties and doubts that only a vacation gives me the chance to look at and deal with. Maybe then I can get from one day to the next without going crazy and keep my child's life "normal". Maybe...

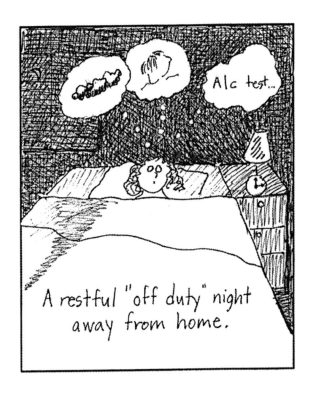

A restful "off duty" night
away from home.

ADDICTED TO CARE GIVING, PART TWO

One part of my journey completed, I crawl into a nice warm bed, turn out the lights and gaze out at the freshly fallen snow. The icy crystals illuminate the night sky as if it were the moon on earth. I gradually fall asleep, relieved that I will not have to get up to check on Byron. Midnight comes, I am up and walking across the room to find Byron. The walls are different, the door is different, and Byron is nowhere to be found. Ah, that's right, I don't have to get up. Back to sleep again.

Two hours later I am up, and again, and again. So much for

rest. My body seems to have memorized my well-practiced schedule of checking him throughout the night. I even have a dream about his A1C test. I dream that the result is 30 and that the doctors are going to take him away from us. The dreams continue.

I don't dream about this stuff when I am with him. So what does all of this mean? At one point during the night, I begin to understand how poorly I have been sleeping for the past few years. I begin to understand why I am so exhausted most of the time, why I am not as patient as I used to be, why I go to bed at 9:00 rather than 11:00, and why I might feel a bit blue now and then. Mostly, I begin to grasp the magnitude of my new job. Being a pancreas is tough work! Still, a real pancreas never sleeps, and at least I get some!

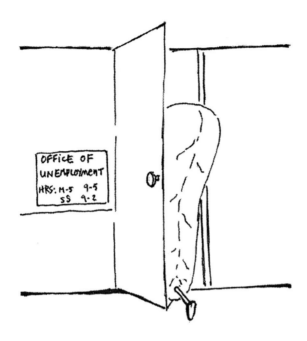

RETIRED PANCREAS LOOKING FOR WORK

As I conclude this book, Byron is in 5th grade, he is almost 11, it has been nearly 5 years since he was diagnosed, and he has taken back a good part of his role as a pancreas. (The pump helped a lot. We like to call it his external pancreas.) During the day, my phone rings less. I don't receive many instant messages alerting me of out of control blood sugars. He no longer has an aid at school. My days are rarely broken up by visits to school to change a pump site or to inject him with insulin. The teachers are calm, the kids are calm, Byron is calm. He accepts where he is, and he is independent. There are still the night checks, but other than that, he is pretty independent. He still asks questions and wants a vacation from his diabetes here and there, but still he is rather independent. Where does this leave me?

I think I have put myself out of a job. I suppose that is the way it is supposed to be. Still, where do you go in life after being a pancreas? Am I semi-retired? Will my job kick back in when he becomes an adolescent? Am I completely retired or is this simply a sabbatical? What title do I have now? What future is there for a has-been pancreas?

Printed in the United States
90822LV00008B/236/A